Snippets of Health

A collection of Healthy Quotes

Dave Farnham

Copyright © 2016 Dave Farnham

ISBN: 1530815630
ISBN-13: 978-1530815630

Also by Dave Farnham

Introduction

There is no shortage of advice on how to keep healthy, whether it's the grossly exaggerated claims for a particular product by the advertising industry or the plethora of pamphlets to be found in a doctor's waiting room. In fact, such an avalanche of advice is so commonplace that we often ignore it, especially as there are numerous conflicting reports in newspapers about what is or isn't healthy. One day we are told to drink coffee to stave off a range of ailments and then a week later the same newspaper warns of the dire dangers of caffeine. So it's hardly surprising that when the press urges us to eat five portions of fruit and vegetables a day we tend to take it with a pinch of salt – which, incidentally, also has health warnings attached to its over-consumption.

By the time we have read the newspapers, watched television programmes about the dangers of sugar, diesel emissions and suntans, and found scare stories about the side effects of almost any medication, we are left with either a sense of impending doom or sheer astonishment that the human race continues to exist.

A hugely profitable industry has developed on the back of our uncertainty about what's healthy and what's not and our search to prevent or cure a vast range of conditions; running alongside conventional medicine, it has a variety of terms: holistic, alternative, homeopathic... Small wonder that, with so many companies claiming to have the answer to health problems (some of which we never realised we had), we're constantly looking for ways to protect ourselves, to avoid an even unhealthier future; it can become quite an obsession.

The suggestions, views and experiences in this book, put forward by both famous and ordinary people, can help you to reach your own conclusions about how to stay healthy.

I wish you the very best of emotional and physical health.

Snippets of Health

"To enjoy good health, to bring true happiness to one's family, to bring peace to all, one must first discipline and control one's own mind. If a man can control his mind he can find the way to Enlightenment, and all wisdom and virtue will naturally come to him."

- Buddha

*

"All mankind... being all equal and independent, no one ought to harm another in his life, health, liberty or possessions."

- John Locke

*

"I've always had a burning desire to help people and make a difference in the world. I didn't know how I could do that in modelling when it can be such a fake world. But my dad told me I could make a difference by being true to myself and teaching people what I've learnt about spirituality, health and nutrition."

- Miranda Kerr

*

"America's health care system is in crisis precisely because we systematically neglect wellness and prevention."

- Tom Harkin

*

"The way you think, the way you behave, the way you eat, can influence your life by 30 to 50 years."

- Deepak Chopra

*

"The groundwork of all happiness is health."

- Leigh Hunt

*

"To enjoy the glow of good health, you must exercise."

- Gene Tunney

*

"The torch relay is an excellent embodiment of all that the Olympic Games have come to symbolise - a celebration of the human spirit. Personally to me, it represents striving to be the best in whatever we do, never giving up despite the odds, and a commitment to health and fitness."

- Lakshmi Mittal

*

"The typical response from people when I tell them I'm

diabetic is, 'Oh, I'm sorry to hear that.' You know, I'm not. I'm a better athlete because of diabetes rather than despite it. I'm more aware of my training, my fitness and more aware of nutrition. I'm more proactive about my health."

- Charlie Kimball

*

"Everybody needs beauty as well as bread, places to play in and pray in, where nature may heal and give strength to body and soul."

- John Muir

*

"I think what it does is it gives me a much broader perspective than the average politician. You know, having walked in those shoes of being hungry and being homeless. The indignities of not getting health care, or waiting in the public hospital, hoping somebody will care for you. Going to sleep with a toothache because you can't go to the dentist."

- Richard Carmona

*

"I think that age as a number is not nearly as important as health. You can be in poor health and be pretty miserable at 40 or 50. If you're in good health, you can enjoy things into your 80s."

- Bob Barker

*

"My health may be better preserved if I exert myself less, but in the end doesn't each person give his life for his calling?"

- Clara Schumann

*

"We are all born with a unique genetic blueprint, which lays out the basic characteristics of our personality as well as our physical health and appearance... And yet, we all know that life experiences do change us."

- Joan D. Vinge

*

"To keep the body in good health is a duty... otherwise we shall not be able to keep our mind strong and clear."

- Buddha

*

"The health effects of air pollution imperil human lives. This fact is well-documented."

- Eddie Bernice Johnson

*

"I love working out. It's my release. I've done it since I've been in the military."

- Robert Irvine

*

"'Tis healthy to be sick sometimes."

- Henry David Thoreau

*

"Being in control of your life and having realistic expectations about your day-to-day challenges are the keys to stress management, which is perhaps the most important ingredient to living a happy, healthy and rewarding life."

- Marilu Henner

*

"America's health care system is neither healthy, caring, nor a system."

- Walter Cronkite

*

"I was born on the other side of the tracks, in public

housing in Brooklyn, New York. My dad never made more than $20,000 a year, and I grew up in a family that lost health insurance. So I was scarred at a young age with understanding what it was like to watch my parents lose access to the American dream."

- Howard Schultz

*

"The greatest of follies is to sacrifice health for any other kind of happiness."

- Arthur Schopenhauer

*

"A healthy attitude is contagious but don't wait to catch it from others. Be a carrier."

- Tom Stoppard

*

"Tobacco is the only industry that produces products to make huge profits and at the same time damage the health and kill their consumers."

- Margaret Chan

*

"A person whose mind is quiet and satisfied in God is in the pathway to health."

- Ellen G. White

*

"Women in particular need to keep an eye on their physical and mental health, because if we're scurrying to and from appointments and errands, we don't have a lot of time to take care of ourselves. We need to do a better job of putting ourselves higher on our own 'to do' list."

- Michelle Obama

*

"As the blessings of health and fortune have a beginning, so they must also find an end. Everything rises but to fall, and increases but to decay."

- Sallust

*

"We should be concerned not only about the health of individual patients, but also the health of our entire society."

- Benjamin Carson

*

"Knowing that we can be loved exactly as we are gives us all the best opportunity for growing into the healthiest of people."

- Fred Rogers

*

"All the money in the world can't buy you back good health."

- Reba McEntire

*

"Did you ever see the customers in health-food stores? They are pale, skinny people who look half dead. In a steak house, you see robust, ruddy people. They're dying, of course, but they look terrific."

- Bill Cosby

*

"The trouble with always trying to preserve the health of the body is that it is so difficult to do without destroying the health of the mind."

- Gilbert K. Chesterton

*

"Perfect freedom is as necessary to the health and vigor of commerce as it is to the health and vigor of citizenship."

- Patrick Henry

*

"Never continue in a job you don't enjoy. If you're happy in what you're doing, you'll like yourself, you'll have inner peace. And if you have that, along with physical health, you will have had more success than you could possibly have imagined."

- Johnny Carson

*

"Man needs difficulties; they are necessary for health."

- Carl Jung

*

"If we could give every individual the right amount of nourishment and exercise, not too little and not too much, we would have found the safest way to health."

- Hippocrates

*

"I know a man who gave up smoking, drinking, sex, and rich food. He was healthy right up to the day he killed himself."

- Johnny Carson

*

"Good health and good sense are two of life's greatest blessings."

- Publilius Syrus

*

"There's nothing more important than our good health -

that's our principal capital asset."

- Arlen Specter

*

"Those who enjoy their own emotionally bad health and who habitually fill their own minds with the rank poisons of suspicion, jealousy and hatred, as a rule take umbrage at those who refuse to do likewise, and they find a perverted relief in trying to denigrate them."

- Johannes Brahms

*

"Time and health are two precious assets that we don't recognize and appreciate until they have been depleted."

- Denis Waitley

*

"Steroids can seem necessary to compete at the highest

levels, and the quick rewards can outweigh the long term consequences to the user's health."

- Howard Berman

*

"As long as man continues to be the ruthless destroyer of lower living beings he will never know health or peace. For as long as men massacre animals, they will kill each other."

- Pythagoras

*

"America has the best doctors, the best nurses, the best hospitals, the best medical technology, the best medical breakthrough medicines in the world. There is absolutely no reason we should not have in this country the best health care in the world."

- Bill Frist

*

"And that means that no matter how we reform health care, we will keep this promise to the American people: If you like your doctor, you will be able to keep your doctor, period. If you like your health care plan, you'll be able to keep your health care plan, period. No one will take it away, no matter what."

- Barack Obama

*

"The essence of global health equity is the idea that something so precious as health might be viewed as a right."

- Paul Farmer

*

"The devil has put a penalty on all things we enjoy in life. Either we suffer in health or we suffer in soul or we get fat."

- Albert Einstein

*

"Liberty is to the collective body, what health is to every individual body. Without health no pleasure can be tasted by man; without liberty, no happiness can be enjoyed by society."

- Henry St. John

*

"Poverty is multidimensional. It extends beyond money incomes to education, health care, political participation and advancement of one's own culture and social organisation."

- Atal Bihari Vajpayee

*

"The health care system is really designed to reward you for being unhealthy. If you are a healthy person and work hard to be healthy, there are no benefits."

- Mike Huckabee

*

"Health consists with temperance alone."

- Alexander Pope

*

"Early to bed and early to rise makes a man healthy, wealthy and wise."

- Benjamin Franklin

*

"The first wealth is health."

- Ralph Waldo Emerson

*

"Healing is a matter of time, but it is sometimes also a matter of opportunity."

- Hippocrates

*

"It is amazing that people who think we cannot afford to pay for doctors, hospitals, and medication somehow think that we can afford to pay for doctors, hospitals, medication and a government bureaucracy to administer it."

- Thomas Sowell

*

"The problem is that everywhere the gas drilling industry goes, a trail of water contamination, air pollution, health concerns and betrayal of basic American civic and community values follows."

- Josh Fox

*

"Well, I think that abstinence has its place as part of a comprehensive health and sex education curriculum. It would be wrong to exclude abstinence from a health curriculum, because there are some potentially very serious ramifications for early sexual activity."

- Kerry Healey

*

"The chief condition on which, life, health and vigor depend, is action. It is by action that an organism develops its faculties, increases its energy, and attains the fulfillment of its destiny."

- Colin Powell

*

"Doing all we can to combat climate change comes with numerous benefits, from reducing pollution and associated health care costs to strengthening and diversifying the economy by shifting to renewable energy, among other measures."

- David Suzuki

*

"If you don't think your anxiety, depression, sadness and stress impact your physical health, think again. All of these emotions trigger chemical reactions in your body, which can lead to inflammation and a weakened immune system. Learn how to cope, sweet friend. There will always be dark days."

- Kris Carr

*

"You don't have to be a wreck. You don't have to be sick. One's aim in life should be to die in good health. Just like a candle that burns out."

- Jeanne Moreau

*

"Health is not a condition of matter, but of Mind."

- Mary Baker Eddy

*

"I have never yet met a healthy person who worried very much about his health, or a really good person who worried much about his own soul."

- John B. S. Haldane

*

"Sleep is that golden chain that ties health and our bodies together."

- Thomas Dekker

*

"I'm not the healthiest, but I am healthy. I'm healthy to the point where there are things that I have to eat that I don't want to eat, but I eat it because I'm enjoying staying alive."

- Bill Cosby

*

"Give a man health and a course to steer, and he'll never stop to trouble about whether he's happy or not."

- George Bernard Shaw

*

"Natural forces within us are the true healers of disease."

- Hippocrates

*

"We have to treat smoking as a major public health issue. We have to reduce the extent to which young people start smoking, and one of the issues is the extent to which display of cigarettes and brands does draw young people into smoking in the first place."

- Andrew Lansley

*

"Think of an economy where people could be an artist or

a photographer or a writer without worrying about keeping their day job in order to have health insurance."

- Nancy Pelosi

*

"A desire to be in charge of our own lives, a need for control, is born in each of us. It is essential to our mental health, and our success, that we take control."

- Robert Foster Bennett

*

"Be careful about reading health books. You may die of a misprint."

- Mark Twain

*

"I just want to be healthy and stay alive and keep my family going and everything and keep my friends going and try to do something so that this world will be peaceful. That is the most ambitious and the most difficult thing, but I'm there trying to do it."

- Yoko Ono

*

"All the evidence that we have indicates that it is reasonable to assume in practically every human being, and certainly in almost every newborn baby, that there is an active will toward health, an impulse towards growth, or towards the actualization."

- Abraham Maslow

*

"I believe that the greatest gift you can give your family and the world is a healthy you."

- Joyce Meyer

*

"Care for life and physical health, with due regard for the needs of others and the common good, is concomitant with respect for human dignity."

- Salvatore J. Cordileone

*

"By themselves, genetically engineered crops will not end hunger or improve health or bolster the economies of struggling countries. They won't save the sight of millions or fortify their bones. But they will certainly help."

- Michael Specter

*

"A library is a place that is a repository of information and gives every citizen equal access to it. That includes health information. And mental health information. It's a community space. It's a place of safety, a haven from the world."

- Neil Gaiman

*

"But the real secret to lifelong good health is actually the opposite: Let your body take care of you."

- Deepak Chopra

*

"When you are young and healthy, it never occurs to you that in a single second your whole life could change."

- Annette Funicello

*

"Hunger and malnutrition have devastating consequences for children and have been linked to low birth weight and birth defects, obesity, mental and physical health problems, and poorer educational outcomes."

- Marian Wright Edelman

*

"If we can get people to focus on fruits and vegetables and more healthy foods, we'll be better in terms of our healthcare situation."

- Tom Vilsack

*

"I'm sure that the standard of public morality we've helped build will force government in Canada to approve complete health insurance."

- Tommy Douglas

*

"Some people are naturally thin, and some are heavier. There is a lot of focus on it, and it can be a lot of pressure for people. But honestly, I think as long as someone is healthy, that is most important."

- Jennifer Lopez

*

"Happiness lies first of all in health."

- George William Curtis

*

"Having good health, being able to breathe and be happy, that's one of the most beautiful gifts. On top of that, I have the gift to play music and make people happy through that. I'm just telling you from my heart, I'm so in love with life."

- Roy Ayers

*

"Hearty laughter is a good way to jog internally without having to go outdoors."

- Norman Cousins

*

"Healthy people are those who live in healthy homes on a healthy diet; in an environment equally fit for birth, growth work, healing, and dying... Healthy people need no bureaucratic interference to mate, give birth, share the human condition and die."

- Ivan Illich

*

"The biggest public health challenge is rebuilding health systems. In other words, if you look at cholera or maternal mortality or tuberculosis in Haiti, they're major problems in Haiti, but the biggest problem is rebuilding systems."

- Paul Farmer

*

"What the public expects and what is healthy for an individual are two very different things."

- Esther Williams

*

"You're in pretty good shape for the shape you are in."

- Dr. Seuss

*

"He who has health, has hope; and he who has hope, has everything."

- Thomas Carlyle

*

"You know, true love really matters, friends really matter, family really matters. Being responsible and disciplined and healthy really matters."

- Courtney Thorne-Smith

*

"Health is the soul that animates all the enjoyments of life, which fade and are tasteless without it."

- Lucius Annaeus Seneca

*

"Seeds and nuts are indispensable for cardiovascular health. The protective properties of nuts against coronary heart disease were first recognized in the early 1990s, and a strong body of literature has followed, confirming these original findings."

- Joel Fuhrman

*

"The biggest mistake people make is to try to lose too much weight too fast."

- Mehmet Oz

*

"It is health that is real wealth and not pieces of gold and silver."

- Mahatma Gandhi

*

"A healthy love life is not and should not be the preserve of those in their 20s and 30s. It's important at all ages."

- Jerry Hall

*

"True silence is the rest of the mind, and is to the spirit what sleep is to the body, nourishment and refreshment."

- William Penn

*

"I have the body of an eighteen year old. I keep it in the fridge."

- Spike Milligan

*

"The wish for healing has always been half of health."

- Lucius Annaeus Seneca

*

"Your body hears everything your mind says."

- Naomi Judd

*

"Older people shouldn't eat health food, they need all the preservatives they can get."

- Robert Orben

*

"True friendship is like sound health; the value of it is seldom known until it is lost."

- Charles Caleb Colton

*

"Look up, laugh loud, talk big, keep the color in your cheek and the fire in your eye, adorn your person, maintain your health, your beauty and your animal spirits."

- William Hazlitt

*

"I support health care for people. I want people well taken care of. But I also want health care that we can afford as a country. I have people and friends closing down their businesses because of Obamacare."

- Donald Trump

*

"I find it a lot healthier for me to be someplace where I can go outside in my bare feet."

- James Taylor

*

"Not necessity, not desire - no, the love of power is the demon of men. Let them have everything - health, food, a place to live, entertainment - they are and remain unhappy and low-spirited: for the demon waits and waits and will be satisfied."

- Friedrich Nietzsche

*

"I'm exhausted trying to stay healthy."

- Steve Yzerman

*

"Learning is the beginning of wealth. Learning is the beginning of health. Learning is the beginning of spirituality. Searching and learning is where the miracle process all begins."

- Jim Rohn

*

"Health is the greatest gift, contentment the greatest
wealth, faithfulness the best relationship."

- Buddha

*

"I have a healthy body, free of the chemicals that once
controlled it."

- Lorna Luft

*

"Our greatest happiness does not depend on the
condition of life in which chance has placed us, but is
always the result of a good conscience, good health,
occupation, and freedom in all just pursuits."

- Thomas Jefferson

*

"Lost wealth may be replaced by industry, lost knowledge by study, lost health by temperance or medicine, but lost time is gone forever."

- Samuel Smiles

*

"At the end of the day, sleep is a barometer of your emotional health. And so if you're not in the right place where you need to be, then you're going to have voices keeping you up at night because you have to work through those issues."

- Mehmet Oz

*

"The health of the people is of supreme importance. All measures looking to their protection against the spread of contagious diseases and to the increase of our sanitary knowledge for such purposes deserve attention of Congress."

- Chester A. Arthur

*

"Pay mind to your own life, your own health, and wholeness. A bleeding heart is of no help to anyone if it bleeds to death."

- Frederick Buechner

*

"I have been very blessed in my life and rewarded with good friends and good health. I am grateful and happy to be able to share this."

- Eric Idle

*

"The foundation of success in life is good health: that is the substratum fortune; it is also the basis of happiness. A person cannot accumulate a fortune very well when he is sick."

- P. T. Barnum

*

"It takes more than just a good looking body. You've got to have the heart and soul to go with it."

- Epictetus

*

"Leave all the afternoon for exercise and recreation, which are as necessary as reading. I will rather say more necessary because health is worth more than learning."

- Thomas Jefferson

*

"Use your health, even to the point of wearing it out. That is what it is for. Spend all you have before you die; do not outlive yourself."

- George Bernard Shaw

*

"If nuclear power plants are safe, let the commerical insurance industry insure them. Until these most expert judges of risk are willing to gamble with their money, I'm not willing to gamble with the health and safety of my family."

- Donna Reed

*

"Health is the vital principle of bliss, and exercise, of health."

- James Thomson

*

"Eventually, competition and adventure wane, and I enter my ibuprofen phase. Tweaky hamstrings and achy knees restrict mileage, but I continue running for health, sanity, and the ritual of a Sunday trail run with like-minded buddies. We discuss the nagging injuries that bedevil us, and remember the good old days when we were kings."

- Don Kardong

*

"Health is the greatest possession. Contentment is the greatest treasure. Confidence is the greatest friend. Non-being is the greatest joy."

- Lao Tzu

*

"I've made a promise to myself to be a 100% healthy person if nothing else."

- Picabo Street

*

"I made a commitment to completely cut out drinking and anything that might hamper me from getting my mind and body together. And the floodgates of goodness have opened upon me - spiritually and financially."

- Denzel Washington

*

"I sit on my duff, smoke cigarettes and watch TV. I'm not exactly a poster girl for healthy living."

- Lexa Doig

*

"Studies have shown that inmate participation in education, vocational and job training, prison work skills development, drug abuse, mental health and other treatment programs, all reduce recidivism, significantly."

- Bobby Scott

*

"There is one consolation in being sick; and that is the possibility that you may recover to a better state than you were ever in before."

- Henry David Thoreau

*

"If you're happy, if you're feeling good, then nothing else matters."

- Robin Wright

*

"I believe that if you're healthy, you're capable of doing everything. There's no one else who can give you health but God, and by being healthy I believe that God is listening to me."

- Pedro Martinez

*

"To be stupid, selfish, and have good health are three requirements for happiness, though if stupidity is lacking, all is lost."

- Gustave Flaubert

*

"Health is the thing that makes you feel that now is the best time of the year."

- Franklin Pierce Adams

*

"It is no measure of health to be well adjusted to a profoundly sick society."

- Jiddu Krishnamurti

*

"Obamacare is not about improved health care or cheaper insurance or better treatment or insuring the uninsured, and it never has been about that. It's about statism. It's about expanding the government. It's about control over the population. It is about everything but health care."

- Rush Limbaugh

*

"As long as your body is healthy and under control and death is distant, try to save your soul; when death is imminent what can you do?"

- Chanakya

*

"If you look at suicides, most of them are connected to depression. And the mental health system just fails them. It's so sad. We know what to do. We just don't do it."

- Rosalynn Carter

*

"I always had a philosophy which I got from my father. He used to say, 'Listen. God gave to you the gift to play football. This is your gift from God. If you take care of your health, if you are in good shape all the time, with your gift from God no one will stop you, but you must be prepared.'"

- Pele

*

"If the childhood obesity epidemic remains unchecked, it will condemn many of our kids to shorter lives, as well as the emotional and financial burdens of poor health."

- Richard Carmona

*

"Health is not valued till sickness comes."

- Thomas Fuller

*

"Calm mind brings inner strength and self-confidence, so that's very important for good health."

- Dalai Lama

*

"Religion is part of the human make-up. It's also part of our cultural and intellectual history. Religion was our first attempt at literature, the texts, our first attempt at cosmology, making sense of where we are in the universe, our first attempt at health care, believing in faith healing, our first attempt at philosophy."

- Christopher Hitchens

*

"When wealth is lost, nothing is lost; when health is lost, something is lost; when character is lost, all is lost."

- Billy Graham

*

"Happiness is nothing more than good health and a bad memory."

- Albert Schweitzer

*

"Besides taking jobs from American workers, illegal immigration creates huge economic burdens on our health care system, our education system, our criminal justice system, our environment, our infrastructure and our public safety."

- Jan C. Ting

*

"It has always been the role of government to help solve problems, including and especially health crises. Obesity is a health epidemic across our country, and we have a responsibility as a government and a society to do all we can to promote good nutrition and healthy eating so we can reverse this alarming trend."

- Richard J. Codey

*

"Treasure the love you receive above all. It will survive long after your good health has vanished."

- Og Mandino

*

"I think the healthy way to live is to make friends with the beast inside oneself, and that means not the beast but the shadow. The dark side of one's nature."

- Anthony Hopkins

*

"Health nuts are going to feel stupid someday, lying in hospitals dying of nothing."

- Redd Foxx

*

"Life is a perspective and for me, if a human being has access to school, clean water, food, proper health care, that is the basis of human rights."

- Gelila Bekele

*

"Investing in health will produce enormous benefits."

- Gro Harlem Brundtland

*

"Without health life is not life; it is only a state of langour and suffering - an image of death."

- Buddha

*

"Soil is a living ecosystem, and is a farmer's most precious asset. A farmer's productive capacity is directly related to the health of his or her soil."

- Howard Warren Buffett

*

"It's no longer a question of staying healthy. It's a question of finding a sickness you like."

- Jackie Mason

*

"Happiness, contentment, the health and growth of the soul, depend, as men have proved over and over again, upon some simple issue, some single turning of the soul."

- George A. Smith

*

"Mr. Speaker, our Nation must no longer be complacent about underage drinking and its alarming consequences. We must bring this national public health crisis out of the shadow and into the bright light of a national priority."

- Lucille Roybal-Allard

*

"My body is like breakfast, lunch, and dinner. I don't think about it, I just have it."

- Arnold Schwarzenegger

*

"You know, all that really matters is that the people you love are happy and healthy. Everything else is just sprinkles on the sundae."

- Paul Walker

*

"Attention to health is life's greatest hindrance."

- Plato

*

"Looking after my health today gives me a better hope for tomorrow."

- Anne Wilson Schaef

*

"A wise man should consider that health is the greatest of human blessings, and learn how by his own thought to derive benefit from his illnesses."

- Hippocrates

*

"It's so important to realize that every time you get upset, it drains your emotional energy. Losing your cool makes you tired. Getting angry a lot messes with your health."

- Joyce Meyer

*

"I entered the health care debate in response to a statement in the United States press in summer 2009 which claimed the National Health Service in Great Britain would have killed me off, were I a British citizen. I felt compelled to make a statement to explain the error."

- Stephen Hawking

*

"But reducing harmful emissions, abating our dependence on foreign oil and developing alternative renewable energy sources have benefits that go beyond environmental health, they improve personal health, enhance national security and encourage our nation's economic viability."

- Jim Clyburn

*

"It's quite amazing to me, as I walk around a supermarket or a health food shop, to observe the number of Fairtrade choices: not just staples such as coffee, tea, fresh fruits and rice, but cocoa and chocolate, herbs and spices, honey, ice cream, and jams."

- Sheherazade Goldsmith

*

"Self-esteem is as important to our well-being as legs are to a table. It is essential for physical and mental health and for happiness."

- Louise Hart

*

"Anytime new insight replaces an old assumption or a fossilized perception is the spring. New understandings sprout, new tolerances appear, and new curiosity draws you to previously dark places. Just as the sun shines earlier and longer in the spring, changes that seemed impossible appear to be possible with each new insight into your own health."

- Gary Zukav

*

"A healthy outside starts from the inside."

- Robert Urich

*

"Healthy people live with their world."

- Anne Wilson Schaef

*

"I became a fanatic about healthy food in 1944."

- Gloria Swanson

*

"I believe that how you feel is very important to how you look - that healthy equals beautiful."

- Victoria Principal

*

"Youth is the spirit of adventure and awakening. It is a time of physical emerging when the body attains the vigor and good health that may ignore the caution of temperance. Youth is a period of timelessness when the horizons of age seem too distant to be noticed."

- Ezra Taft Benson

*

"God can cause opportunity to find you. He has unexpected blessings where you suddenly meet the right person, or suddenly your health improves, or suddenly you're able to pay off your house. That's God shifting things in your favor."

- Joel Osteen

*

"The winners in life treat their body as if it were a magnificent spacecraft that gives them the finest transportation and endurance for their lives."

- Denis Waitley

*

"Contrary to popular belief, I don't spend a whole lot of time following soccer. But as I have traveled around the world to better understand global development and health, I've learned that soccer is truly universal. No matter where I go, that's what kids are playing. That's what people are talking about."

- Bill Gates

*

"I feel pretty good. My body actually looks like an old banana, but it's fine."

- Mike Piazza

*

"Many kids come out of college, they have a credit card and a diploma. They don't know how to buy a house or a car or health insurance or life insurance. They do not know basic microeconomics."

- Jesse Jackson

*

"The average, healthy, well-adjusted adult gets up at seven-thirty in the morning feeling just plain terrible."

- Jean Kerr

*

"The power of community to create health is far greater than any physician, clinic or hospital."

- Mark Hyman

*

"Rest when you're weary. Refresh and renew yourself, your body, your mind, your spirit. Then get back to work."

- Ralph Marston

*

"The minute anyone's getting anxious I say, You must eat and you must sleep. They're the two vital elements for a healthy life."

- Francesca Annis

*

"If we get our self-esteem from superficial places, from

our popularity, appearance, business success, financial situation, health, any of these, we will be disappointed, because no one can guarantee that we'll have them tomorrow."

- Kathy Ireland

*

"Quit worrying about your health. It will go away."

- Robert Orben

*

"If workers are more insecure, that's very 'healthy' for the society, because if workers are insecure, they won't ask for wages, they won't go on strike, they won't call for benefits; they'll serve the masters gladly and passively. And that's optimal for corporations' economic health."

- Noam Chomsky

*

"It was the labor movement that helped secure so much of what we take for granted today. The 40-hour work week, the minimum wage, family leave, health insurance, Social Security, Medicare, retirement plans. The cornerstones of the middle-class security all bear the union label."

- Barack Obama

*

"The rise of childhood obesity has placed the health of an entire generation at risk."

- Tom Vilsack

*

"I'm healthy as can be - not an ache or a pain. A lot of my prayer is thanking the Lord that I am healthy. I pray for long life and good health."

- Joel Osteen

*

"Illegal immigration costs taxpayers $45 billion a year in health care, education, and incarceration expenses."

- Ric Keller

*

"The ingredients of health and long life, are great temperance, open air, easy labor, and little care."

- Philip Sidney

*

"Every day I wake up and I lay in bed counting my blessings and saying my prayers for how fortunate I am to have great fans and health and family."

- Luke Bryan

*

"If Obamacare is allowed to stand - and Congress is allowed to make the purchase of government-endorsed health insurance compulsory - there will be no meaningful limit on Washington's reach into the lives of the American people. That is certainly not what the Founders intended."

- John Cornyn

*

"Capital is reckless of the health or length of life of the laborer, unless under compulsion from society."

- Karl Marx

*

"When the Nobel award came my way, it also gave me an opportunity to do something immediate and practical about my old obsessions, including literacy, basic health care and gender equity, aimed specifically at India and Bangladesh."

- Amartya Sen

*

"You cannot have maternal health without reproductive health. And reproductive health includes contraception and family planning and access to legal, safe abortion."

- Hillary Clinton

*

"We can make a commitment to promote vegetables and fruits and whole grains on every part of every menu. We can make portion sizes smaller and emphasize quality over quantity. And we can help create a culture - imagine this - where our kids ask for healthy options instead of resisting them."

- Michelle Obama

*

"True security is based on people's welfare - on a thriving economy, on strong public health and education programmes, and on fundamental respect for our common humanity. Development, peace, disarmament, reconciliation and justice are not separate from security; they help to underpin it."

- Ban Ki-moon

*

"I eat really healthy, and if I'm tired, I take a nap."

- Casper Van Dien

*

"The art of healing comes from nature, not from the physician. Therefore the physician must start from nature, with an open mind."

- Paracelsus

*

"A man is not rightly conditioned until he is a happy, healthy, and prosperous being; and happiness, health, and prosperity are the result of a harmonious adjustment of the inner with the outer of the man with his surroundings."

- James Allen

*

"Money doesn't mean anything to me. I've made a lot of money, but I want to enjoy life and not stress myself building my bank account. I give lots away and live simply, mostly out of a suitcase in hotels. We all know that good health is much more important."

- Keanu Reeves

*

"We don't come to Canada for our health. We can think of other ways of enjoying ourselves."

- Prince Philip

*

"The healthy man does not torture others - generally it is the tortured who turn into torturers."

- Carl Jung

*

"Breast cancer alone kills some 458,000 people each year, according to the World Health Organization, mainly in low- and middle-income countries. It has got to be a priority to ensure that more women can access gene testing and lifesaving preventive treatment, whatever their means and background, wherever they live."

- Angelina Jolie

*

"Antibiotics are a very serious public health problem for us, and it's getting worse. Resistant microbes outstrip new antibiotics. It's an ongoing problem. It's not like we can fix it, and it's over. We have to fight continued resistance with a continual pipeline of new antibiotics and continue with the perpetual challenge."

- Anthony Fauci

*

"You see people who have been very heavy in their life who have taken that body, trimmed it down, firmed it up through discipline, exercise and being able to say no. Eating properly, that all comes into it."

- Mike Ditka

*

"What can be added to the happiness of a man who is in health, out of debt, and has a clear conscience?"

- Adam Smith

*

"Vaccines are the most cost-effective health care interventions there are. A dollar spent on a childhood vaccination not only helps save a life, but greatly reduces spending on future healthcare."

- Ezekiel Emanuel

*

"People who don't know how to keep themselves healthy ought to have the decency to get themselves buried, and not waste time about it."

- Henrik Ibsen

*

"My trust in God flows out of the experience of His loving me, day in and day out, whether the day is stormy or fair, whether I'm sick or in good health, whether I'm in a state of grace or disgrace. He comes to me where I live and loves me as I am."

- Brennan Manning

*

"Cheerfulness is the best promoter of health and is as friendly to the mind as to the body."

- Joseph Addison

*

"I really believe the only way to stay healthy is to eat properly, get your rest and exercise. If you don't exercise and do the other two, I still don't think it's going to help you that much."

- Mike Ditka

*

"I stand before you a totally healthy person."

- Melissa Etheridge

*

"Saving our planet, lifting people out of poverty, advancing economic growth... these are one and the same fight. We must connect the dots between climate change, water scarcity, energy shortages, global health, food security and women's empowerment. Solutions to one problem must be solutions for all."

- Ban Ki-moon

*

"My personal goals are to be happy, healthy and to be surrounded by loved ones."

- Kiana Tom

*

"A healthy human environment is one in which we try to make sense of our limits, of the accidents that can always befall us and the passage of time which inexorably changes us."

- Rowan Williams

*

"The body is a sacred garment."

- Martha Graham

*

"Family, nature and health all go together."

- Olivia Newton-John

*

"Good health is not something we can buy. However, it can be an extremely valuable savings account."

- Anne Wilson Schaef

*

"Faith and prayer are the vitamins of the soul; man cannot live in health without them."

- Mahalia Jackson

*

"The only way to keep your health is to eat what you don't want, drink what you don't like, and do what you'd rather not."

- Mark Twain

*

"Most Christian 'believers' tend to echo the cultural prejudices and worldviews of the dominant group in their country, with only a minority revealing any real transformation of attitudes or consciousness. It has been true of slavery and racism, classism and consumerism and issues of immigration and health care for the poor."

- Richard Rohr

*

"It's better to be healthy alone than sick with someone else."

- Phil McGraw

*

"A good job is more than just a paycheck. A good job fosters independence and discipline, and contributes to the health of the community. A good job is a means to provide for the health and welfare of your family, to own a home, and save for retirement."

- James H. Douglas, Jr.